# THE COMPLETE AFIB DIET COOKBOOK FOR BEGINNERS

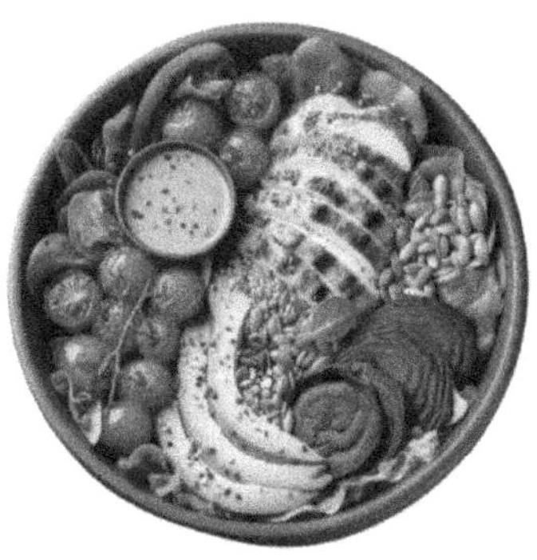

Unlocking the Power of the AFIB Diet to Enhance Heart Health, Boost Energy, and Achieve Natural Weight Balance

Tina Feldman

# Table of Contents

# Introduction

**What is the AFIB Diet?**

The AFIB (Anti-Inflammatory, Balanced, and Energizing) Diet is a revolutionary approach to nutrition designed to optimize health and well-being by focusing on three key principles: combating inflammation, achieving a balance of essential nutrients, and promoting sustained energy levels.

1. **Anti-Inflammatory:**
   The foundation of the AFBI Diet is its emphasis on combating inflammation in the body. Chronic inflammation is linked to various health issues, including heart disease, arthritis, and autoimmune disorders. By incorporating anti-inflammatory foods such as fatty fish, leafy greens, berries, and nuts, the AFIB Diet aims to reduce inflammation and support overall health.

2. **Balanced Nutrition:**
   The AFIB Diet recognizes the importance of a well-rounded and balanced diet. It encourages the consumption of a variety of nutrient-dense foods, including lean proteins, whole grains, fruits, and vegetables. This balance ensures that individuals receive the necessary vitamins, minerals, and other essential nutrients for optimal health and functioning.

3. **Energizing Foods:**
   Sustained energy is crucial for maintaining an active and vibrant lifestyle. The AFIB Diet promotes the consumption of foods that provide a steady release of energy throughout the day. Complex carbohydrates, healthy fats, and proteins are strategically included to prevent energy crashes and maintain a consistent level of vitality.

By combining these three principles, the AFIB Diet not only supports physical health but also contributes to mental well-being. The cookbook for beginners takes these concepts and translates them into practical, delicious recipes that are easy to follow, making the AFIB Diet accessible to individuals at any stage of their wellness journey.

## Benefits of the AFBI Diet

The AFIB (Anti-Inflammatory, Balanced, and Energizing) Diet offers a multitude of benefits that contribute to overall health and well-being. Here are some of the key advantages:

**Inflammation Reduction:**
The AFBI Diet is specifically designed to combat chronic inflammation, which is associated with numerous health issues. By incorporating anti-inflammatory foods, individuals may experience a reduction in inflammation, potentially alleviating symptoms of conditions such as arthritis and inflammatory bowel diseases.
Improved Heart Health:

The emphasis on heart-healthy foods, such as fatty fish rich in omega-3 fatty acids, helps lower cholesterol levels and supports cardiovascular health. This can contribute to a reduced risk of heart disease and related complications.

**Weight Management:**
The AFBI Diet promotes a balanced and nutrient-dense approach to eating, which can aid in weight management. By providing the body with essential nutrients, individuals may experience better control over cravings and achieve sustainable weight loss or maintenance.

**Steady Energy Levels:**
Through the inclusion of complex carbohydrates, lean proteins, and healthy fats, the AFBI Diet supports consistent energy levels throughout the day. This can enhance productivity, mental clarity, and overall vitality.

**Improved Digestive Health:**
The emphasis on fiber-rich foods, such as fruits, vegetables, and whole grains, supports a healthy digestive system. This can alleviate issues like constipation and promote a balanced gut microbiome.

**Enhanced Mental Well-being:**
Nutrient-dense foods play a crucial role in brain health. The AFBI Diet includes foods rich in antioxidants and essential nutrients that support cognitive function, potentially reducing the risk of

cognitive decline and improving overall mental well-being.

**Boosted Immune System:**
Many foods recommended in the AFBI Diet, such as fruits and vegetables, are rich in vitamins and minerals that support a robust immune system. This can help the body defend against infections and illnesses.

**Reduced Risk of Chronic Diseases:**
By addressing inflammation and promoting overall health, the AFBI Diet may contribute to a decreased risk of chronic diseases, including diabetes, certain cancers, and neurodegenerative conditions.

**Balanced Nutrition for All Ages:**
The AFBI Diet is adaptable for people of all ages and life stages. It provides a balanced approach to nutrition, ensuring that individuals receive the essential nutrients required for growth, development, and maintenance of health throughout their lives.

**Delicious and Sustainable Eating Habits:**
The AFBI Diet encourages the consumption of a variety of flavorful and satisfying foods, making it an enjoyable and sustainable way of eating. This can lead to long-term adherence and lifestyle changes.

# Getting Started with AFBI: Essential Tips for Beginners

Embarking on the AFBI (Anti-Inflammatory, Balanced, and Energizing) Diet journey can be an exciting and transformative experience for beginners. Here are essential tips to help you get started and make the most out of your AFBI Diet adventure:

**Educate Yourself:**
Take the time to understand the core principles of the AFBI Diet. Familiarize yourself with anti-inflammatory foods, the importance of balanced nutrition, and the role of energizing foods in maintaining vitality. Knowledge is a powerful tool on your wellness journey.

**Plan and Prep:**
Planning and preparation are key to success. Outline your meals for the week, create a shopping list, and dedicate time to prep ingredients. Having nutritious options readily available reduces the temptation to opt for less healthy choices.

**Explore AFBI-Approved Foods:**
Discover the diverse array of foods that fit the AFBI criteria. This includes anti-inflammatory options like berries, fatty fish, and leafy greens; balanced nutrition from lean proteins, whole grains, and vegetables; and energizing foods such as nuts, seeds, and complex carbohydrates.

**Gradual Transition:**
Transitioning to a new way of eating can be overwhelming. Consider making gradual changes to allow your taste buds and habits to adjust. Start by incorporating one or two AFBI-approved meals a day and gradually increase as you become more comfortable.

**Hydration Matters:**
Adequate hydration is crucial for overall health. Water helps flush out toxins and supports bodily functions. Make water your primary beverage and limit the intake of sugary or caffeinated drinks.

**Mindful Eating:**
Practice mindful eating by savoring each bite and paying attention to hunger and fullness cues. This helps develop a healthier relationship with food and promotes better digestion.

**Experiment with Recipes:**
The AFBI Diet doesn't mean sacrificing flavor. Explore a variety of recipes that align with the principles of the diet. Experiment with herbs and spices to enhance the taste of your meals, making your culinary journey enjoyable and satisfying.

**Listen to Your Body:**
Pay attention to how your body responds to different foods. Everyone is unique, and what works for one person may not work for another. Adjust your food choices based on how your body feels and responds.

Stay Consistent:

Consistency is key to experiencing the full benefits of the AFBI Diet. While occasional indulgences are normal, strive to maintain a consistent approach to your eating habits to maximize the positive impact on your health.

**Seek Support:**
Share your AFBI Diet journey with friends, family, or online communities. Having a support system can provide motivation, accountability, and a platform to exchange tips and recipe ideas.
Remember, the AFBI Diet is not just a short-term plan; it's a lifestyle change aimed at promoting long-term health and well-being. Approach it with curiosity, an open mind, and a commitment to nurturing your body with the best possible nutrition.

# Part 1

## AFBI Fundamentals

Understanding Macronutrients: Protein, Fat, Carbs

Understanding macronutrients—protein, fat, and carbohydrates—is fundamental to the success of the AFBI (Anti-Inflammatory, Balanced, and Energizing) Diet. Each macronutrient plays a crucial role in supporting overall health and well-being. Here's an in-depth exploration of these essential components:

**Protein:**

Function: Proteins are the building blocks of the body. They play a vital role in the growth, repair, and maintenance of tissues, organs, and muscles.

Sources: Include lean meats, poultry, fish, eggs, dairy products, legumes, tofu, and plant-based protein sources like quinoa and lentils.

AFBI Focus: Opt for lean protein sources to minimize saturated fat intake. Fatty fish rich in omega-3 fatty acids, such as salmon, align with the anti-inflammatory aspect of the diet.

**Fat:**

Function: Dietary fats are essential for various bodily functions, including hormone production, absorption of fat-soluble vitamins (A, D, E, K), and providing a long-lasting source of energy.

Sources: Healthy fats are found in avocados, nuts, seeds, olive oil, and fatty fish. Limit saturated and trans fats found in processed foods and red meat.

AFBI Focus: Prioritize sources of unsaturated fats, particularly omega-3 fatty acids. These fats have anti-inflammatory properties and can be found in fatty fish, flaxseeds, and walnuts.

**Carbohydrates:**

Function: Carbohydrates are the body's primary source of energy. They are crucial for brain function and provide fuel for physical activities.

Sources: Whole grains (brown rice, quinoa, oats), fruits, vegetables, legumes, and starchy vegetables like sweet potatoes.

AFBI Focus: Choose complex carbohydrates with a low glycemic index to support sustained energy levels and minimize inflammation. Fiber-rich options, like fruits and vegetables, contribute to digestive health.

Understanding the balance of these macronutrients is key to achieving the goals of the AFBI Diet

Balancing Act: The AFBI Diet encourages a balanced distribution of macronutrients to ensure that the body receives the right proportion of protein, fats, and carbohydrates for optimal function.

Portion Control: Pay attention to portion sizes to prevent overconsumption and maintain a healthy weight. The AFBI Diet emphasizes quality over quantity.

Whole Foods Emphasis: Whenever possible, choose whole, unprocessed foods over refined options. Whole foods provide a broader spectrum of nutrients and align with the anti-inflammatory and balanced nature of the diet.

Individualization: Adjust the macronutrient ratio based on individual needs and goals. Some may thrive on a slightly higher protein intake, while others may benefit from a more carbohydrate-centric approach.

## Building Balanced Plates: AFBI Macro Ratios Explained

Building balanced plates is a fundamental aspect of the AFBI (Anti-Inflammatory, Balanced, and Energizing) Diet, and understanding the macro ratios is crucial for optimizing health. The goal is to create meals that provide a harmonious balance of macronutrients—protein, fat, and carbohydrates. Here's a detailed explanation of the AFBI macro ratios:

**Protein:**
Role in Balanced Plates: Protein is a crucial component of balanced plates as it supports muscle maintenance, repairs tissues, and provides a sense of satiety, preventing overeating.

Recommended Ratio: Aim for approximately 20-30% of your total daily caloric intake to come from protein sources. This ensures an adequate supply for bodily functions without excessive consumption.
Plate Examples: Include lean protein sources like grilled chicken, fish, tofu, or legumes as the central element of your plate.

**Fat:**
Role in Balanced Plates: Healthy fats contribute to sustained energy, support nutrient absorption, and provide a feeling of fullness.
Recommended Ratio: About 25-35% of your daily caloric intake should come from healthy fats. Prioritize sources like avocados, nuts, seeds, and olive oil.
Plate Examples: Incorporate a moderate amount of healthy fats by drizzling olive oil on salads, adding avocado to your meal, or including a handful of nuts.

**Carbohydrates:**
Role in Balanced Plates: Complex carbohydrates are the primary energy source, supporting brain function and physical activities.
Recommended Ratio: Aim for approximately 45-55% of your total daily caloric intake to come from complex carbohydrates. Choose whole grains, fruits, vegetables, and legumes.
Plate Examples: Fill the remaining portion of your plate with colorful vegetables, a serving of whole grains, or a side of sweet potatoes to provide a well-rounded carbohydrate component.

**Fiber:**
Importance in AFBI Diet: While not a macronutrient, fiber is essential for digestive health, helps regulate blood sugar, and contributes to a feeling of fullness. Incorporating Fiber: Opt for whole, fiber-rich foods like fruits, vegetables, whole grains, and legumes. Ensure that each meal contains a good source of dietary fiber to enhance the anti-inflammatory and balanced aspects of the diet.

**Hydration:**
Supporting Nutrient Absorption: Adequate hydration is crucial for nutrient absorption and overall health. Water should be the primary beverage, supporting the principles of the AFBI Diet.
Hydration Tips: Drink water throughout the day, and consider herbal teas or infused water for added flavor without added sugars.

## Approved Foods for Each Macronutrient Group

**Protein Sources:**
4.  Chicken breast
5.  Turkey
6.  Salmon
7.  Tofu
8.  Greek yogurt
9.  Eggs
10. Lentils
11. Chickpeas

12. Quinoa
13. Cottage cheese
14. Shrimp
15. Grass-fed beef
16. Cod
17. Edamame
18. Bison
19. Mackerel
20. Almonds
21. Tempeh
22. Chia seeds
23. Greek yogurt

**Healthy Fat Sources:**
1. Avocado
2. Olive oil
3. Walnuts
4. Flaxseeds
5. Chia seeds
6. Almonds
7. Salmon
8. Coconut oil
9. Pumpkin seeds
10. Dark chocolate (in moderation)
11. Sunflower seeds
12. Cashews
13. Hazelnuts
14. Brazil nuts
15. Macadamia nuts
16. Sesame oil
17. Pecans
18. Nut butters (almond, peanut, or cashew)

19. Hemp seeds
20. Fatty fish like mackerel or sardines

## Complex Carbohydrate Sources:

1. Sweet potatoes
2. Quinoa
3. Brown rice
4. Oats
5. Barley
6. Farro
7. Bulgur
8. Buckwheat
9. Millet
10. Whole grain pasta
11. Whole grain bread
12. Legumes (black beans, kidney beans, chickpeas)
13. Lentils
14. Peas
15. Brussels sprouts
16. Blueberries
17. Strawberries
18. Apples
19. Oranges
20. Cherries

## Fruits and Vegetables:

1. Spinach
2. Kale
3. Broccoli
4. Cauliflower
5. Carrots

6. Bell peppers
7. Tomatoes
8. Cucumbers
9. Zucchini
10. Asparagus
11. Mangoes
12. Pineapple
13. Papaya
14. Berries (blueberries, strawberries, raspberries)
15. Watermelon
16. Grapefruit
17. Pomegranate
18. Kiwi
19. Bananas
20. Oranges

**Dairy and Dairy Alternatives:**
1. Greek yogurt
2. Cottage cheese
3. Almond milk
4. Coconut milk
5. Cashew milk
6. Plain yogurt
7. Kefir
8. Feta cheese
9. Mozzarella cheese
10. Parmesan cheese
11. Goat cheese
12. Ricotta cheese
13. Swiss cheese
14. Provolone cheese

15. Gouda cheese
16. Brie cheese
17. Unsweetened soy milk
18. Plain kefir
19. Skyr
20. Grass-fed butter (in moderation)

## 14-Days meal plan

Day 1: Anti-Inflammatory Salmon Bowl
Ingredients:
Salmon fillet
Quinoa
Spinach
Cherry tomatoes
Avocado
Olive oil, lemon, and herbs for dressing

**Preparation:**
Cook quinoa according to package instructions.
Pan-sear salmon with olive oil.
Assemble a bowl with quinoa, spinach, cherry tomatoes, avocado, and salmon.
Drizzle with a dressing made of olive oil, lemon juice, and herbs.
Prep Time: 25 minutes
Calories: Approximately 450 calories

Day 2: Energizing Breakfast Smoothie
Ingredients:
Greek yogurt

Banana
Spinach
Almond butter
Almond milk
Chia seeds

**Preparation:**
Blend all ingredients until smooth.
Pour into a glass and enjoy.
Prep Time: 10 minutes
Calories: Approximately 350 calories

Day 3: Balanced Quinoa Salad
Ingredients:
Quinoa
Chickpeas
Cucumber
Red bell pepper
Feta cheese
Olive oil and balsamic vinegar for dressing

**Preparation:**
Cook quinoa and let it cool.
Mix quinoa with chickpeas, cucumber, red bell pepper, and feta cheese.
Drizzle with olive oil and balsamic vinegar.
Prep Time: 20 minutes
Calories: Approximately 400 calories

Day 4: Anti-Inflammatory Chicken Stir-Fry
Ingredients:
Chicken breast

Broccoli
Bell peppers
Ginger and garlic for seasoning
Brown rice

**Preparation:**
Cook brown rice according to package instructions.
Stir-fry chicken with broccoli and bell peppers,
seasoned with ginger and garlic.
Serve over brown rice.
Prep Time: 30 minutes
Calories: Approximately 500 calories

Day 5: Energizing Berry Salad with Grilled Tofu
Ingredients:
Mixed berries (blueberries, strawberries, raspberries)
Tofu
Mixed greens
Walnuts
Balsamic vinaigrette

**Preparation:**
Grill tofu until golden.
Toss mixed greens with berries, walnuts, and grilled
tofu.
Drizzle with balsamic vinaigrette.
Prep Time: 25 minutes
Calories: Approximately 380 calories

Day 6: Balanced Veggie Omelette
Ingredients:
Eggs

Spinach
Tomatoes
Mushrooms
Feta cheese
Olive oil

**Preparation:**
Whisk eggs and pour into a heated skillet.
Add spinach, tomatoes, mushrooms, and feta cheese.
Cook until eggs are set.
Prep Time: 15 minutes
Calories: Approximately 320 calories
Day 7: Anti-Inflammatory Lentil Soup
Ingredients:
Lentils
Carrots
Celery
Onion
Garlic
Turmeric and cumin for seasoning

**Preparation:**
Cook lentils with carrots, celery, onion, and garlic.
Season with turmeric and cumin.
Prep Time: 35 minutes
Calories: Approximately 280 calories

Day 8: Energizing Acai Bowl
Ingredients:
Acai puree
Banana
Mixed berries

Granola
Chia seeds
Almond butter

**Preparation:**
Blend acai puree with banana and mixed berries.
Top with granola, chia seeds, and a drizzle of almond
butter.
Prep Time: 15 minutes
Calories: Approximately 420 calories


Day 9: Balanced Turkey and Veggie Skewers
Ingredients:
Turkey breast
Zucchini
Cherry tomatoes
Bell peppers
Olive oil and herbs for seasoning
Quinoa

**Preparation:**
Cut turkey and veggies into skewer-sized pieces.
Season with olive oil and herbs.
Grill until cooked, serve with quinoa.
Prep Time: 25 minutes
Calories: Approximately 480 calories

Day 10: Anti-Inflammatory Stuffed Bell Peppers
Ingredients:
Ground turkey

Quinoa
Black beans
Corn
Tomatoes
Cumin and paprika for seasoning

**Preparation:**
Cook quinoa and brown ground turkey.
Mix with black beans, corn, tomatoes, and season
with cumin and paprika.
Stuff bell peppers and bake until tender.
Prep Time: 40 minutes
Calories: Approximately 370 calories

Day 11: Energizing Green Smoothie Bowl
Ingredients:
Spinach
Kale
Pineapple
Banana
Coconut water
Hemp seeds

**Preparation:**
Blend spinach, kale, pineapple, banana, and coconut
water until smooth.
Pour into a bowl and top with hemp seeds.
Prep Time: 10 minutes
Calories: Approximately 350 calories

Day 12: Balanced Shrimp and Quinoa Stir-Fry
Ingredients:

Shrimp
Quinoa
Broccoli
Snap peas
Carrots
Soy sauce and ginger for seasoning

**Preparation:**
Cook quinoa and set aside.
Stir-fry shrimp with broccoli, snap peas, and carrots,
seasoned with soy sauce and ginger.
Serve over quinoa.
Prep Time: 30 minutes
Calories: Approximately 420 calories
Day 13: Anti-Inflammatory Grilled Vegetable Salad
with Chicken
Ingredients:
Grilled chicken breast
Eggplant
Zucchini
Red onion
Cherry tomatoes
Balsamic vinaigrette

**Preparation:**
Grill chicken and vegetables.
Toss together with cherry tomatoes and drizzle with
balsamic vinaigrette.
Prep Time: 35 minutes
Calories: Approximately 480 calories

Day 14: Energizing Chia Pudding Parfait

Ingredients:
Chia seeds
Almond milk
Greek yogurt
Mixed berries
Granola

**Preparation:**
Mix chia seeds with almond milk and let it sit overnight.
Layer chia pudding with Greek yogurt, mixed berries, and granola.
Prep Time: 10 minutes (plus overnight soaking)
Calories: Approximately 350 calories

# Part 2

## AFBI Recipes

## Breakfast:

Energizing Breakfast Smoothie Bowl
Ingredients:
Acai puree
Banana
Mixed berries
Granola
Chia seeds
Almond butter

**Preparation:**

Blend acai puree with banana and mixed berries.
Top with granola, chia seeds, and a drizzle of almond butter.
Prep Time: 10 minutes
Calories: Approximately 420 calories

Balanced Veggie Omelette
Ingredients:
Eggs
Spinach
Tomatoes
Mushrooms
Feta cheese
Olive oil

**Preparation:**
Whisk eggs and pour into a heated skillet.
Add spinach, tomatoes, mushrooms, and feta cheese.
Cook until eggs are set.
Prep Time: 15 minutes
Calories: Approximately 320 calories

Anti-Inflammatory Chia Seed Pudding
Ingredients:
Chia seeds
Almond milk
Greek yogurt
Mixed berries
Honey (optional)

**Preparation:**
Mix chia seeds with almond milk and Greek yogurt.
Let it sit in the refrigerator overnight.
Top with mixed berries and a drizzle of honey if desired.
Prep Time: 10 minutes (plus overnight soaking)
Calories: Approximately 300 calories

Energizing Greek Yogurt Parfait
Ingredients:
Greek yogurt
Mixed berries
Granola
Almonds
Honey

**Preparation:**
Layer Greek yogurt with mixed berries, granola, and almonds.
Drizzle with honey.
Prep Time: 5 minutes
Calories: Approximately 350 calories

Balanced Avocado Toast with Poached Egg
Ingredients:
Whole grain bread
Avocado
Poached egg
Cherry tomatoes
Olive oil

**Preparation:**
Toast whole grain bread.
Mash avocado and spread it on the toast.
Top with a poached egg, cherry tomatoes, and a drizzle of olive oil.
Prep Time: 15 minutes
Calories: Approximately 380 calories

Anti-Inflammatory Overnight Oats
Ingredients:
Rolled oats
Almond milk
Greek yogurt
Blueberries
Almond butter

**Preparation:**
Mix rolled oats with almond milk and Greek yogurt.
Add blueberries and a dollop of almond butter.
Let it sit in the refrigerator overnight.
Prep Time: 10 minutes (plus overnight soaking)
Calories: Approximately 340 calories

Energizing Quinoa Breakfast Bowl
Ingredients:
Cooked quinoa
Mixed berries
Greek yogurt
Almonds

Maple syrup (optional)

**Preparation:**
Combine cooked quinoa with mixed berries and Greek yogurt.
Top with almonds and a drizzle of maple syrup if desired.
Prep Time: 15 minutes
Calories: Approximately 400 calories

Balanced Spinach and Feta Breakfast Wrap
Ingredients:
Whole grain tortilla
Eggs
Spinach
Feta cheese
Cherry tomatoes
Olive oil

**Preparation:**
Scramble eggs and cook with spinach.
Fill a whole grain tortilla with the egg mixture, feta cheese, and cherry tomatoes.
Drizzle with olive oil.
Prep Time: 20 minutes
Calories: Approximately 340 calories

Anti-Inflammatory Smoked Salmon Bagel
Ingredients:
Whole grain bagel
Smoked salmon

Cream cheese (optional)
Cucumber slices
Dill

**Preparation:**
Toast the whole grain bagel.
Spread with cream cheese if desired.
Top with smoked salmon, cucumber slices, and fresh dill.
Prep Time: 10 minutes
Calories: Approximately 380 calories

Energizing Banana and Almond Butter Toast
Ingredients:
Whole grain bread
Banana slices
Almond butter
Chia seeds

**Preparation:**
Toast whole grain bread.
Spread almond butter on the toast and top with banana slices.
Sprinkle it with chia seeds.
Prep Time: 5 minutes
Calories: Approximately 320 calories

## Lunch

Anti-Inflammatory Grilled Chicken Salad
Ingredients:

Grilled chicken breast
Mixed greens (kale, spinach, arugula)
Cherry tomatoes
Avocado
Olive oil and balsamic vinegar for dressing

**Preparation:**
Grill chicken and slice into strips.
Toss mixed greens with cherry tomatoes and sliced avocado.
Drizzle with olive oil and balsamic vinegar.
Prep Time: 20 minutes
Calories: Approximately 450 calories

Balanced Quinoa and Vegetable Stir-Fry
Ingredients:
Quinoa
Broccoli
Carrots
Snap peas
Tofu or chicken
Soy sauce and ginger for seasoning
**Preparation:**
Cook quinoa according to package instructions.
Stir-fry tofu or chicken with broccoli, carrots, and snap peas, seasoned with soy sauce and ginger.
Serve over cooked quinoa.
Prep Time: 30 minutes
Calories: Approximately 480 calories

Energizing Chickpea and Spinach Wrap
Ingredients:

Whole grain wrap
Chickpeas
Spinach
Cherry tomatoes
Hummus

**Preparation:**
Warm the whole grain wrap.
Fill with chickpeas, spinach, cherry tomatoes, and a
spread of hummus.
Prep Time: 15 minutes
Calories: Approximately 380 calories
Anti-Inflammatory Lentil and Vegetable Soup

Ingredients:
Lentils
Carrots
Celery
Onion
Garlic
Turmeric and cumin for seasoning

**Preparation:**
Cook lentils with carrots, celery, onion, and garlic.
Season with turmeric and cumin.
Prep Time: 35 minutes
Calories: Approximately 280 calories

Balanced Turkey and Quinoa Stuffed Bell Peppers
Ingredients:
Bell peppers

Ground turkey
Quinoa
Black beans
Corn
Tomatoes

**Preparation:**
Cook quinoa and brown ground turkey.
Mix with black beans, corn, tomatoes.
Stuff bell peppers and bake until tender.
Prep Time: 40 minutes
Calories: Approximately 370 calories

Energizing Sweet Potato and Chickpea Buddha Bowl
Ingredients:
Sweet potatoes
Chickpeas
Broccoli
Avocado
Tahini dressing

**Preparation:**
Roast sweet potatoes, chickpeas, and broccoli.
Assemble a bowl with the roasted ingredients and sliced avocado.
Drizzle with tahini dressing.
Prep Time: 30 minutes
Calories: Approximately 420 calories

Anti-Inflammatory Salmon and Quinoa Bowl
Ingredients:
Salmon fillet
Quinoa
Spinach
Cherry tomatoes
Avocado
Olive oil, lemon, and herbs for dressing

**Preparation:**
Cook quinoa according to package instructions.
Pan-sear salmon with olive oil.
Assemble a bowl with quinoa, spinach, cherry tomatoes, avocado, and salmon.
Drizzle with a dressing made of olive oil, lemon juice, and herbs.
Prep Time: 25 minutes
Calories: Approximately 450 calories

Balanced Shrimp and Vegetable Brown Rice Bowl
Ingredients:
Shrimp
Brown rice
Broccoli
Snap peas
Carrots
Soy sauce and garlic for seasoning

**Preparation:**
Cook brown rice according to package instructions.
Stir-fry shrimp with broccoli, snap peas, and carrots, seasoned with soy sauce and garlic.

Serve over brown rice.
Prep Time: 30 minutes
Calories: Approximately 500 calories

Energizing Caprese Salad with Grilled Chicken
Ingredients:
Grilled chicken breast
Tomatoes
Fresh mozzarella
Basil leaves
Balsamic glaze

**Preparation:**
Grill chicken breast.
Slice tomatoes and fresh mozzarella.
Arrange in layers with basil leaves and drizzle with
balsamic glaze.
Prep Time: 20 minutes
Calories: Approximately 380 calories

Anti-Inflammatory Mediterranean Chickpea Salad
Ingredients:
Chickpeas
Cucumber
Cherry tomatoes
Kalamata olives
Feta cheese
Olive oil and lemon dressing

**Preparation:**
Rinse and drain chickpeas.

Combine chickpeas with diced cucumber, cherry tomatoes, Kalamata olives, and crumbled feta cheese.
Drizzle with olive oil and lemon dressing.
Prep Time: 15 minutes
Calories: Approximately 360 calories

## Dinner

Anti-Inflammatory Baked Salmon with Roasted Vegetables
Ingredients:
Salmon fillet
Sweet potatoes
Brussels sprouts
Olive oil, lemon, and herbs for seasoning

**Preparation:**
Season salmon with olive oil, lemon, and herbs.
Roast sweet potatoes and Brussels sprouts alongside the salmon.
Prep Time: 30 minutes
Calories: Approximately 400 calories

Balanced Turkey and Vegetable Stir-Fry
Ingredients:
Ground turkey
Bell peppers
Broccoli
Snow peas
Quinoa
Soy sauce and ginger for seasoning

**Preparation:**
Brown ground turkey in a skillet.
Stir-fry bell peppers, broccoli, and snow peas, seasoned with soy sauce and ginger.
Serve over cooked quinoa.
Prep Time: 25 minutes
Calories: Approximately 480 calories

Energizing Veggie and Tofu Curry
Ingredients:
Tofu
Cauliflower
Spinach
Coconut milk
Curry spices (turmeric, cumin, coriander)

**Preparation:**
Pan-fry tofu until golden.
Simmer cauliflower and spinach in coconut milk with curry spices.
Add tofu and let simmer until vegetables are tender.
Prep Time: 35 minutes
Calories: Approximately 350 calories

Anti-Inflammatory Grilled Chicken with Quinoa Salad
Ingredients:
Grilled chicken breast

Quinoa
Cucumber
Tomatoes
Feta cheese
Olive oil and lemon dressing

**Preparation:**
Grill chicken breast and slice into strips.
Cook quinoa and let it cool.
Toss quinoa with diced cucumber, tomatoes, feta cheese, and a dressing made of olive oil and lemon.
Prep Time: 30 minutes
Calories: Approximately 420 calories

Balanced Lentil and Vegetable Stuffed Peppers
Ingredients:
Lentils
Bell peppers
Zucchini
Onion
Garlic
Tomato sauce

**Preparation:**
Cook lentils with diced zucchini, onion, and garlic.
Stuff bell peppers with the lentil mixture and bake with tomato sauce.
Prep Time: 40 minutes
Calories: Approximately 370 calories
Energizing Quinoa and Black Bean Bowl
Ingredients:
Quinoa

Black beans
Corn
Avocado
Lime and cilantro for seasoning

**Preparation:**
Cook quinoa according to package instructions.
Mix quinoa with black beans, corn, and diced avocado.
Season with lime and cilantro.
Prep Time: 20 minutes
Calories: Approximately 380 calories

Anti-Inflammatory Chickpea and Spinach Curry
Ingredients:
Chickpeas
Spinach
Tomatoes
Coconut milk
Curry spices (turmeric, cumin, coriander)

**Preparation:**
Simmer chickpeas, spinach, and diced tomatoes in coconut milk with curry spices.
Allow to simmer until flavors meld.
Prep Time: 30 minutes
Calories: Approximately 350 calories

Balanced Shrimp and Vegetable Skewers with Quinoa
Ingredients:

Shrimp
Zucchini
Cherry tomatoes
Quinoa
Olive oil and herbs for seasoning

**Preparation:**
Cook quinoa according to package instructions.
Thread shrimp, zucchini, and cherry tomatoes onto skewers.
Grill or bake skewers, seasoned with olive oil and herbs.
Prep Time: 35 minutes
Calories: Approximately 500 calories

Energizing Sweet Potato and Black Bean Enchiladas
Ingredients:
Sweet potatoes
Black beans
Corn tortillas
Enchilada sauce
Avocado

**Preparation:**
Roast sweet potatoes and mix with black beans.
Fill corn tortillas with the sweet potato and black bean mixture.
Bake with enchilada sauce and serve with sliced avocado.
Prep Time: 45 minutes
Calories: Approximately 420 calories

Anti-Inflammatory Mediterranean Grilled Veggie Salad
Ingredients:
Eggplant
Zucchini
Red bell peppers
Cherry tomatoes
Feta cheese
Olive oil and balsamic vinegar for dressing

**Preparation:**
Grill eggplant, zucchini, and red bell peppers until tender.
Toss with cherry tomatoes and crumbled feta cheese.
Drizzle with olive oil and balsamic vinegar.
Prep Time: 30 minutes
Calories: Approximately 380 calories

## Snacks

Energy-Boosting Greek Yogurt Parfait
Ingredients:
Greek yogurt
Mixed berries
Almonds
Honey

**Preparation:**
Layer Greek yogurt with mixed berries and almonds.
Drizzle with honey.
Prep Time: 5 minutes
Calories: Approximately 250 calories

Balanced Hummus and Veggie Sticks
Ingredients:
Hummus
Carrot sticks
Cucumber slices
Bell pepper strips

**Preparation:**
Slice vegetables into sticks.
Dip in hummus.
Prep Time: 10 minutes
Calories: Approximately 180 calories

Anti-Inflammatory Avocado Toast Bites
Ingredients:
Whole grain crackers
Avocado
Cherry tomatoes

Chia seeds
**Preparation:**
Spread mashed avocado on whole grain crackers.
Top with sliced cherry tomatoes and a sprinkle of chia seeds.
Prep Time: 15 minutes
Calories: Approximately 200 calories

Energizing Trail Mix
Ingredients:
Almonds
Walnuts
Dried blueberries
Pumpkin seeds
Dark chocolate chips (in moderation)

**Preparation:**
Mix all ingredients in a bowl.
Portion into small snack bags.
Prep Time: 5 minutes
Calories: Approximately 200 calories

Balanced Apple Slices with Almond Butter
Ingredients:
Apple slices
Almond butter
Cinnamon (optional)

**Preparation:**
Spread almond butter on apple slices.
Sprinkle with cinnamon if desired.
Prep Time: 5 minutes

Calories: Approximately 150 calories

Anti-Inflammatory Roasted Chickpeas
Ingredients:
Chickpeas
Olive oil
Turmeric and cumin
Sea salt

**Preparation:**
Rinse and dry chickpeas.
Toss with olive oil, turmeric, cumin, and a pinch of
sea salt.
Roast until crispy.
Prep Time: 40 minutes (including roasting time)
Calories: Approximately 150 calories

**Energizing Berry and Nut Smoothie**
Ingredients:
Mixed berries
Almond milk
Greek yogurt
Almonds
Chia seeds

**Preparation:**
Blend mixed berries, almond milk, and Greek yogurt
until smooth.
Top with chopped almonds and chia seeds.
Prep Time: 10 minutes
Calories: Approximately 220 calories

Balanced Whole Grain Toast with Cottage Cheese
Ingredients:
Whole grain bread
Cottage cheese
Sliced strawberries
Honey

**Preparation:**
Toast whole grain bread.
Spread cottage cheese on the toast and top with sliced
strawberries.
Drizzle with honey.
Prep Time: 10 minutes
Calories: Approximately 180 calories

Anti-Inflammatory Veggie Roll-Ups
Ingredients:
Zucchini slices
Hummus
Turkey or chicken slices

**Preparation:**
Spread hummus on zucchini slices.
Place a slice of turkey or chicken on top and roll up.
Prep Time: 15 minutes
Calories: Approximately 160 calories

Energizing Banana and Almond Smoothie
Ingredients:

Banana
Almond milk
Almond butter
Spinach
**Preparation:**
Blend banana, almond milk, almond butter, and spinach until smooth.
Prep Time: 5 minutes
Calories: Approximately 220 calories

## Smoothies

Energizing Green Goddess Smoothie
Ingredients:
Spinach
Pineapple chunks
Banana
Greek yogurt
Almond milk

**Preparation:**
Blend spinach, pineapple chunks, banana, Greek yogurt, and almond milk until smooth.
Prep Time: 5 minutes
Calories: Approximately 220 calories

Balanced Berry Bliss Smoothie
Ingredients:
Mixed berries (strawberries, blueberries, raspberries)
Quinoa flakes
Almond butter
Greek yogurt

Coconut water

**Preparation:**
Blend mixed berries, quinoa flakes, almond butter, Greek yogurt, and coconut water until smooth.
Prep Time: 7 minutes
Calories: Approximately 250 calories

Anti-Inflammatory Turmeric Mango Smoothie
Ingredients:
Mango chunks
Pineapple chunks
Turmeric powder
Ginger
Coconut milk

**Preparation:**
Blend mango chunks, pineapple chunks, turmeric powder, ginger, and coconut milk until smooth.
Prep Time: 6 minutes
Calories: Approximately 230 calories

Energizing Citrus Sunshine Smoothie
Ingredients:
Oranges (peeled and segmented)
Banana
Carrot (peeled and chopped)
Greek yogurt
Orange juice

**Preparation:**

Blend oranges, banana, carrot, Greek yogurt, and orange juice until smooth.
Prep Time: 8 minutes
Calories: Approximately 210 calories

Balanced Almond Joy Smoothie
Ingredients:
Almond milk
Almonds
Dark chocolate chips (in moderation)
Coconut flakes
Banana

**Preparation:**
Blend almond milk, almonds, dark chocolate chips, coconut flakes, and banana until smooth.
Prep Time: 6 minutes
Calories: Approximately 240 calories

## Desserts

Anti-Inflammatory Berry Chia Seed Pudding
Ingredients:
Chia seeds
Almond milk
Mixed berries (blueberries, strawberries, raspberries)
Honey (optional)

**Preparation:**

Mix chia seeds with almond milk and let it sit in the refrigerator for a few hours or overnight.
Layer the chia pudding with mixed berries.
Drizzle with honey if desired.
Prep Time: 4 hours (including chilling time)
Calories: Approximately 180 calories


Balanced Dark Chocolate-Dipped Almond Bites
Ingredients:
Almonds
Dark chocolate (70% cocoa or higher)
Sea salt

**Preparation:**
Melt dark chocolate in a microwave or on a stovetop.
Dip each almond into the melted chocolate.
Sprinkle with a pinch of sea salt.
Allow to cool and harden.
Prep Time: 20 minutes
Calories: Approximately 160 calories

Energizing Grilled Pineapple with Cinnamon
Ingredients:
Pineapple slices
Cinnamon
Greek yogurt (optional)

**Preparation:**
Grill pineapple slices until they develop grill marks.
Sprinkle with cinnamon.

Serve with a dollop of Greek yogurt if desired.
Prep Time: 15 minutes
Calories: Approximately 130 calories


Anti-Inflammatory Baked Apple with Almond Crumble
Ingredients:
Apples (cored and sliced)
Almond flour
Coconut oil
Cinnamon
Maple syrup (optional)

**Preparation:**
Toss apple slices with a sprinkle of cinnamon.
In a separate bowl, mix almond flour, melted coconut oil, and a touch of maple syrup.
Place apple slices in a baking dish and top with the almond crumble mixture.
Bake until apples are tender.
Prep Time: 30 minutes
Calories: Approximately 200 calories

Balanced Coconut and Berry Ice Cream
Ingredients:
Frozen mixed berries
Coconut milk

Unsweetened shredded coconut

**Preparation:**
Blend frozen berries with coconut milk until smooth.
Stir in shredded coconut.
Transfer the mixture to an airtight container and freeze until firm.
Prep Time: 10 minutes (plus freezing time)
Calories: Approximately 150 calories


# Part 3


# AFBI Lifestyle

## Staying Hydrated: Importance of Water and Tips for Increased Intake

Certainly! Staying hydrated is a crucial aspect of maintaining a healthy and balanced lifestyle, especially in the context of the AFBI (Anti-Inflammatory, Balanced, and Energizing) lifestyle. Here are details about the importance of water and tips for increased intake:

**Importance of Water in the AFBI Lifestyle:**
**Cellular Function:**

Water is essential for various cellular processes, ensuring that cells function optimally. This is vital for overall health and well-being.

Detoxification:
Adequate hydration supports the body's natural detoxification processes, helping to eliminate waste and toxins. This aligns with the anti-inflammatory principles of the AFBI lifestyle.

Joint Health:
Water plays a key role in maintaining joint health by lubricating joints and facilitating smooth movement. This is particularly important for individuals following an active and balanced lifestyle.

Digestive Health:
Proper hydration aids in digestion and nutrient absorption. It helps prevent constipation and supports a healthy gastrointestinal system, contributing to the overall balance promoted by the AFBI lifestyle.

Temperature Regulation:
Water is crucial for regulating body temperature, especially during physical activities. This is essential for individuals incorporating energizing exercises into their routine.

Cognitive Function:
Dehydration can negatively impact cognitive function, including concentration and memory. Staying hydrated supports mental clarity, aligning with the AFBI lifestyle's emphasis on overall well-being.

## Tips for Increased Water Intake in the AFBI Lifestyle:

Set a Schedule:
Establish a routine for drinking water throughout the day. This can include having a glass of water upon waking up, before meals, and between meals.

Flavor with Natural Additions:
Enhance the taste of water with natural additions like lemon slices, cucumber, or mint. This can make hydration more enjoyable, encouraging increased intake.
Use Hydration Apps:
Utilize smartphone apps designed to remind you to drink water at regular intervals. These apps can be customized to suit your preferences and activity levels.

Invest in a Quality Water Bottle:
Carry a reusable water bottle with you throughout the day. Having a convenient and aesthetically pleasing bottle can make it more likely that you'll consistently reach for it.

Monitor Urine Color:
Pay attention to the color of your urine. Pale yellow or straw-colored urine generally indicates proper hydration, while dark yellow may suggest dehydration. Use this as a visual guide.

Pair with Meals:

Drink water with meals to aid in digestion. This also helps create a balanced approach to hydration, ensuring you're not consuming large amounts at once.

Herbal Teas and Infusions:
Include herbal teas or infusions in your hydration routine. This provides variety while contributing to your overall fluid intake.

Set Hydration Goals:
Establish daily hydration goals based on your activity level, climate, and individual needs. This can serve as a benchmark to ensure you are consistently meeting your hydration needs.

Listen to Your Body:
Pay attention to your body's signals for thirst. Often, thirst is a reliable indicator that it's time to rehydrate. Respond promptly to these signals.

Hydrate Before, During, and After Exercise:
Exercise increases the body's water requirements. Stay ahead of dehydration by drinking water before, during, and after physical activity, aligning with the energizing aspect of the AFBI lifestyle.

## Exercise & Movement: Finding Activities You Enjoy for a Sustainable Lifestyle

Integrating exercise and movement into your daily routine is a key component of the AFBI (Anti-

Inflammatory, Balanced, and Energizing) lifestyle. Here's a guide on how to find activities you enjoy for a sustainable and enjoyable approach to fitness:

## Importance of Exercise in the AFBI Lifestyle: Anti-Inflammatory Benefits:

Regular physical activity has been linked to reduced inflammation in the body. This aligns with the anti-inflammatory focus of the AFBI lifestyle, promoting overall health.

Balanced Well-Being:
Exercise contributes to a balanced lifestyle by improving mood, reducing stress, and enhancing mental well-being. It complements the holistic approach of the AFBI lifestyle.

Energizing Effect:
Engaging in physical activity boosts energy levels and vitality. It aligns with the energizing aspect of the AFBI lifestyle, promoting an active and fulfilling life.

Joint and Muscle Health:
Regular movement supports joint flexibility and muscle strength. This is essential for individuals following an active lifestyle, ensuring they maintain mobility and strength.

Enhanced Metabolism:
Exercise plays a role in maintaining a healthy weight and supporting metabolism. This contributes to the overall balance promoted by the AFBI lifestyle.
Finding Activities You Enjoy:

Explore Variety:
Experiment with a variety of activities to discover what resonates with you. This could include yoga, hiking, swimming, cycling, dancing, or team sports. The AFBI lifestyle encourages diversity in activities for a well-rounded approach.

Consider Preferences:
Reflect on activities you enjoyed in the past or those that align with your interests. If you enjoy being outdoors, activities like hiking or gardening may be appealing.

Social Engagement:
Choose activities that allow for social interaction. Joining a sports club, group fitness classes, or partnering with a workout buddy can make exercise more enjoyable and sustainable.

Mind-Body Connection:
Incorporate activities that promote a mind-body connection, such as yoga or tai chi. These practices align with the balanced and holistic principles of the AFBI lifestyle.

Make it Fun:
Opt for activities that feel like play rather than a chore. Whether it's dancing to your favorite music, playing a sport you love, or participating in recreational activities, making it fun enhances sustainability.

Adapt to Preferences:
Adapt your exercise routine to suit your preferences and lifestyle. If you prefer short, intense workouts, consider high-intensity interval training (HIIT). If you enjoy a more relaxed pace, activities like walking or gentle stretching may be preferable.

Set Realistic Goals:
Set achievable and realistic fitness goals. This could include gradually increasing the duration or intensity of your workouts. Sustainable progress is key to maintaining a consistent exercise routine.

Incorporate Functional Movement:
Focus on activities that have practical applications in daily life. This could involve functional movements like squats, lunges, and core exercises, contributing to the balanced and practical nature of the AFBI lifestyle.

Listen to Your Body:
Pay attention to how your body responds to different activities. Choose exercises that leave you feeling

invigorated rather than exhausted, emphasizing the energizing aspect of the AFBI lifestyle.

Mix and Match:
Combine different activities to keep things interesting. This not only prevents boredom but also ensures that you engage various muscle groups, promoting overall fitness.

## Creating a Sustainable Routine:
Consistency Over Intensity:
Prioritize consistency in your exercise routine over intensity. Regular, moderate activity is more sustainable and aligns with the balanced approach of the AFBI lifestyle.

Schedule Regular Breaks:
Allow for rest days and recovery. Overtraining can lead to burnout, whereas a well-paced routine supports long-term adherence.

Adapt to Changes:
Be adaptable and open to modifying your routine as circumstances change. This flexibility is crucial for sustaining a long-term commitment to exercise.

Celebrate Achievements:
Celebrate your fitness achievements, whether they're big or small. Recognizing progress is motivating and contributes to the positive, balanced mindset of the AFBI lifestyle.

Integrate Movement Into Daily Life:
Look for opportunities to move throughout the day. This could involve taking the stairs, walking during breaks, or incorporating short bursts of activity into your routine.

# Meal Prep & Planning: Strategies for Saving Time and Making Healthy Choices Easy

Meal prep and planning are essential components of the AFBI (Anti-Inflammatory, Balanced, and Energizing) lifestyle, making it easier to save time and maintain healthy eating habits. Here's a comprehensive guide on strategies for effective meal prep and planning:

## Importance of Meal Prep in the AFBI Lifestyle: Nutritional Consistency:

Meal prep ensures that you have access to balanced and nutritious meals consistently. This aligns with the principles of the AFBI lifestyle, emphasizing the importance of nutrient-dense foods.

Time Efficiency:
Planning and preparing meals in advance save time during busy periods. This allows for a more efficient and sustainable approach to maintaining a healthy lifestyle.

Portion Control:
Preparing meals in advance enables better control over portion sizes. This contributes to balanced nutrition and supports weight management, a key aspect of the AFBI lifestyle.

Reduced Stress:

Having meals ready to go reduces the stress associated with daily food decisions. It promotes a sense of control and organization, supporting overall well-being.

Financial Savings:
Meal prepping can lead to cost savings as it minimizes the need for impulsive and potentially less healthy food choices. This aligns with the balanced and mindful spending aspects of the AFBI lifestyle. Strategies for Effective Meal Prep and Planning:

Create a Weekly Menu:
Plan your meals for the week ahead. Consider a variety of nutrient-dense foods, incorporating different colors, textures, and flavors to align with the AFBI lifestyle's emphasis on balance.

Batch Cooking:
Prepare larger quantities of staple foods like grains, proteins, and vegetables. This simplifies assembling meals throughout the week, saving time and ensuring variety.

Utilize a Meal Prep Day:
Designate a specific day for meal prep. Use this time to chop vegetables, cook proteins, and assemble components that can be easily combined for quick and healthy meals.

Invest in Quality Containers:
Choose durable, portion-sized containers to store your meals. This not only helps with portion control but also ensures that your food stays fresh.

Mindful Ingredient Choices:
Select ingredients with the AFBI lifestyle in mind. Opt for whole grains, lean proteins, and a colorful array of fruits and vegetables to maximize nutritional value.

Incorporate Variety:
Plan for variety within your meals. Rotate protein sources, include different vegetables, and experiment with various herbs and spices to keep meals interesting and aligned with the AFBI lifestyle's emphasis on diversity.

Include Snacks:
Don't forget to prep healthy snacks. Having pre-portioned snacks readily available helps avoid reaching for less nutritious options when hunger strikes.

Prep Breakfasts and Lunches:
Focus on preparing breakfasts and lunches, as these are often the busiest times of the day. Overnight oats, smoothie packs, and pre-assembled salads are convenient options.

Use Freezer-Friendly Meals:

Prepare meals that can be frozen for later use. This provides flexibility and ensures a variety of options are available, aligning with the AFBI lifestyle's adaptability.

Stay Organized:
Keep a well-organized kitchen. Label containers with the date and contents, and arrange ingredients for easy access. This promotes efficiency during meal prep.

Plan for Leftovers:
Plan meals with leftovers in mind. Cook extra portions that can be repurposed into different meals, reducing the need for constant cooking.

Stay Mindful of Seasonal Produce:
Incorporate seasonal produce into your meal plans. This not only enhances flavor but also ensures a diverse and fresh approach to your nutrition, supporting the AFBI lifestyle's emphasis on whole foods.

Create a Grocery List:
Before shopping, create a detailed grocery list based on your weekly menu. This minimizes impulse purchases and ensures you have all the necessary ingredients.

Rotate Recipes:
Keep a repertoire of go-to recipes but also experiment with new ones. This prevents mealtime

monotony, contributing to the enjoyable and balanced nature of the AFBI lifestyle.

Adapt to Lifestyle Changes:
Be flexible and adapt your meal prep routine to changes in your schedule or lifestyle. This ensures that meal prep remains a sustainable practice.

## Sample Grocery List: Stocking Your Pantry with AFBI Staples

**Fresh Produce:**
1. Spinach
2. Kale
3. Broccoli
4. Bell peppers (various colors)
5. Avocado
6. Berries (blueberries, strawberries, raspberries)
7. Tomatoes
8. Cucumbers
9. Sweet potatoes
10. Lemons
11. Proteins:
12. Lean chicken breast
13. Salmon
14. Turkey (ground or whole)
15. Eggs
16. Tofu
17. Greek yogurt
18. Lentils
19. Chickpeas

**Whole Grains:**
1. Quinoa
2. Brown rice
3. Oats

4. Whole wheat pasta
5. Farro
6. Barley

**Healthy Fats:**
1. Olive oil
2. Coconut oil
3. Nuts (almonds, walnuts)
4. Seeds (flaxseeds, chia seeds)
5. Nut butter (almond or peanut butter)
6. Flaxseed oil

**Dairy and Alternatives:**
1. Low-fat or plant-based milk (almond, soy, or coconut)
2. Feta cheese
3. Parmesan cheese
4. Cottage cheese (low-fat or plant-based)

**Herbs and Spices:**
1. Turmeric
2. Ginger
3. Cumin
4. Coriander
5. Basil
6. Oregano
7. Rosemary
8. Garlic powder
9. Cinnamon

**Canned Goods:**
1. Tomatoes (diced, crushed)

2. Tomato paste
3. Black beans
4. Chickpeas
5. Lentils
6. Tuna (in water)
7. Low-sodium vegetable or chicken broth

## Condiments:
1. Dijon mustard
2. Balsamic vinegar
3. Olive tapenade
4. Hummus
5. Salsa (without added sugars)
6. Tahini

## Baking Essentials:
1. Whole wheat flour
2. Almond flour
3. Baking powder
4. Baking soda
5. Honey or maple syrup (for sweetening in moderation)

## Frozen Foods:
1. Mixed berries (for smoothies)
2. Broccoli florets
3. Spinach
4. Peas

## Beverages:
1. Green tea
2. Herbal teas (chamomile, peppermint)

3.  Sparkling water

**Snacks:**
1.  Rice cakes
2.  Air-popped popcorn
3.  Raw vegetables (carrot sticks, celery)
4.  Hummus for dipping

**Grilled Items:**
1.  Grilled chicken
2.  Grilled salmon
3.  Grilled vegetables (zucchini, eggplant)

**Miscellaneous:**
1.  Dark chocolate (70% cocoa or higher)
2.  Coconut flakes
3.  Unsweetened almond milk for beverages and cooking
4.  Rolled oats for breakfast or baking
5.  Low-sodium soy sauce or tamari

# Kitchen Essentials: Tools and Equipment for Easy AFBI Cooking

Creating a well-equipped kitchen is essential for easy and enjoyable cooking that aligns with the principles of the AFBI (Anti-Inflammatory, Balanced, and Energizing) lifestyle. Here's a guide to essential tools and equipment that will make your AFBI cooking experience more efficient and enjoyable:

## Cookware

Quality Chef's Knife:
Invest in a sharp, high-quality chef's knife. It's a versatile tool for chopping, slicing, and dicing a variety of ingredients.

Cutting Boards:
Have separate cutting boards for vegetables, fruits, and proteins to prevent cross-contamination. Choose boards made of durable and easy-to-clean materials.

Non-Stick Skillet:
A non-stick skillet is great for cooking with less oil and for quick, healthy sautéing. Look for a durable, non-toxic option.

Stainless Steel Pots and Pans:
Stainless steel cookware is durable, distributes heat evenly, and is easy to clean. Consider a variety of sizes for different cooking needs.

Baking Sheets and Pans:

Have a variety of baking sheets and pans for roasting vegetables, preparing sheet pan meals, and baking healthy treats.

Cast Iron Skillet:
A cast iron skillet is excellent for even heat distribution and can be used for a variety of cooking methods, including stovetop and oven cooking.
Kitchen Tools:

Wooden Spoons and Spatulas:
Wooden utensils are gentle on cookware and won't scratch non-stick surfaces. They're perfect for stirring, flipping, and serving.

Tongs:
Tongs are versatile for flipping, turning, and serving food. Look for ones with a non-slip grip.

Vegetable Peeler:
Make preparing fruits and vegetables quick and easy with a reliable vegetable peeler.

Box Grater:
A box grater is useful for grating vegetables, cheese, and other ingredients. Look for one with various grating options.

Microplane Zester:

Perfect for zesting citrus fruits, grating ginger, and adding flavorful touches to your dishes.
Measuring Cups and Spoons:

Precision is key in cooking. Invest in accurate measuring cups and spoons for precise ingredient amounts.

Colander:
A colander is essential for draining pasta, rinsing vegetables, and washing fruits.

## Appliances

Blender:
A high-quality blender is essential for smoothies, soups, and sauces. Look for one with various speed settings and durable blades.

Food Processor:
A food processor is versatile for chopping, slicing, and pureeing ingredients. It's a time-saving tool for meal prep.

Slow Cooker or Instant Pot:
These appliances are excellent for easy and convenient cooking. They are ideal for preparing stews, soups, and one-pot meals with minimal effort.

Juicer:
If you enjoy fresh juices, a juicer can be a valuable addition to your kitchen.

Storage:

Glass Storage Containers:
Use glass containers for storing leftovers and meal prepped ingredients. They are safe for reheating and are more environmentally friendly than plastic.

Mason Jars:
Mason jars are versatile for storing salads, overnight oats, and homemade sauces.
Miscellaneous:

Kitchen Scale:
For precise portion control and accurate measurements, a kitchen scale is invaluable.

Oven Mitts and Pot Holders:
Ensure safety in the kitchen with heat-resistant oven mitts and pot holders.

Kitchen Timer:
Keep track of cooking times to prevent overcooking or burning.

Reusable Cooking Liners:
Non-stick reusable cooking liners are a great alternative to parchment paper and reduce waste.

# Tips for Choosing Kitchen Essentials

Quality Over Quantity:
Invest in durable, high-quality items that will last.

Multi-Functional Tools:
Look for tools and equipment that can perform multiple functions to maximize utility in a small kitchen.

Storage Space:
Consider your kitchen space and storage options when selecting kitchen tools and equipment.

Easy to Clean:
Opt for items that are easy to clean and maintain for hassle-free cooking.

By equipping your kitchen with these essentials, you'll be well-prepared to embrace the AFBI lifestyle with easy, nutritious, and delicious cooking

# Recipe Substitutions: Adapting Recipes to Fit Your Preferences and Dietary Needs

Adapting recipes to fit your preferences and dietary needs is a skill that aligns seamlessly with the AFBI (Anti-Inflammatory, Balanced, and Energizing) lifestyle. Whether you have specific dietary restrictions, preferences, or are simply looking to enhance the nutritional value of your meals, here's a guide to making thoughtful and health-conscious recipe substitutions:

1. Flour Substitutes:
    1. Almond Flour: Replace traditional wheat flour with almond flour for a gluten-free and nutrient-dense alternative in baking.
    2. Coconut Flour: A low-carb and gluten-free option, coconut flour works well in baked goods.

2. Sugar Substitutes:
    1. Maple Syrup or Honey: Use these natural sweeteners as alternatives to refined sugar.
    2. Stevia or Monk Fruit: For those seeking zero-calorie options, these sweeteners can replace sugar in recipes.

3. Cooking Oils:
    1. Olive Oil: Substitute vegetable oils with heart-healthy olive oil for its anti-inflammatory properties.

2. Coconut Oil: Adds a distinct flavor and is a stable option for cooking at higher temperatures.

4. Dairy Alternatives:
   1. Almond Milk, Coconut Milk, or Oat Milk: Replace cow's milk with these plant-based alternatives for a dairy-free option.
   2. Nutritional Yeast: Provides a cheesy flavor in vegan or dairy-free dishes.

5. Protein Sources:
   1. Tofu or Tempeh: Ideal substitutes for meat, offering plant-based protein.
   2. Quinoa or Lentils: For a protein boost, use these alternatives in place of rice or pasta.

6. Grain Alternatives:
   1. Cauliflower Rice: A low-carb alternative to traditional rice.
   2. Zucchini Noodles (Zoodles): Replace pasta with spiralized zucchini for a lighter dish.

7. Salt Substitutes:
   1. Herbs and Spices: Enhance flavor with herbs like basil, oregano, and thyme, or spices like turmeric and cumin, reducing the need for excess salt.
   2. Sea Salt or Himalayan Pink Salt: Opt for these mineral-rich alternatives over standard table salt.

8. Egg Replacements:
   1. Flaxseed or Chia Seed Eggs: Mix ground flaxseeds or chia seeds with water to create a gel-like consistency, serving as an egg substitute.
   2. Applesauce or Mashed Banana: Use these for moisture and binding in baking.

9. Pasta Alternatives:
   1. Whole Wheat or Brown Rice Pasta: Substitute traditional pasta with whole grains for added fiber.
   2. Spaghetti Squash: Create noodle-like strands by roasting spaghetti squash for a low-carb option.

10. Nutritional Boosts:
   1. Turmeric or Ginger: Add anti-inflammatory properties to dishes for health benefits.
   2. Chia Seeds or Flaxseeds: Increase omega-3 fatty acids, fiber, and texture in recipes.

11. Fresh Herbs and Citrus:
   1. Basil, Cilantro, or Parsley: Infuse dishes with fresh flavors and antioxidants.
   2. Lemon or Lime Juice: Brighten up dishes with citrus for a burst of flavor.

12. Mindful Portion Control:
   - Use Smaller Plates: Create visual cues for portion control by using smaller plates, promoting mindful eating.

**Tips for Successful Substitutions**
1. Experiment Gradually: Make one substitution at a time to understand its impact on flavor and texture.
2. Consider Flavor Profiles: Choose substitutions that complement the overall flavor profile of the dish.
3. Be Mindful of Allergies: When substituting, consider any allergies or sensitivities.
4. Adapting recipes to fit your preferences and dietary needs not only enhances the nutritional value of your meals but also allows you to tailor your food to the principles of the AFBI lifestyle. Enjoy the creative process of experimenting with substitutions, and find the perfect balance that suits your taste and health goals.

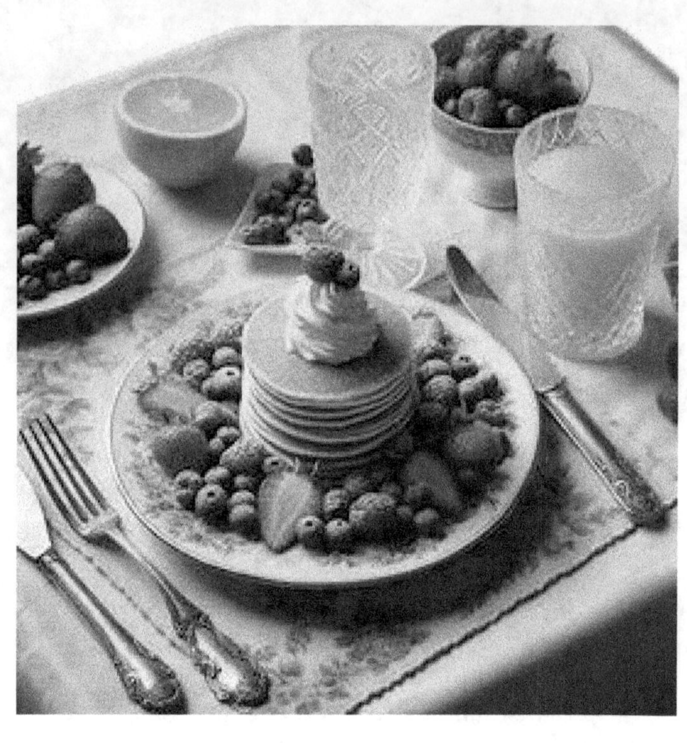

# Conclusion

In conclusion, the AFBI (Anti-Inflammatory, Balanced, and Energizing) Diet Cookbook for Beginners is more than just a collection of recipes; it's a journey towards a healthier, more vibrant lifestyle. As we've explored the foundations of the AFBI diet, delved into the benefits, and provided a comprehensive guide to delicious and nutritious recipes, it becomes clear that this cookbook is a valuable companion for anyone seeking a mindful and balanced approach to nutrition.

The AFBI Diet Cookbook empowers beginners with knowledge about anti-inflammatory ingredients, balanced macronutrient ratios, and energizing food choices. By understanding the significance of each component, readers can make informed decisions about their dietary habits, fostering not only physical well-being but also a harmonious relationship with food.

The cookbook embraces diversity, offering a wide array of recipes suitable for various tastes and preferences. From breakfast to dinner, snacks to desserts, each dish is crafted with a focus on nourishment and flavor. The inclusion of detailed nutritional information ensures that individuals can make choices aligned with their dietary goals, promoting a sense of control over their health journey.

Moreover, the cookbook encourages culinary creativity, inspiring readers to adapt recipes to their liking and dietary needs. With insights into ingredient substitutions and practical kitchen tips, beginners can confidently experiment with flavors while staying true to the principles of the AFBI lifestyle.

As users embark on the 14-day meal plan, they not only experience the convenience of structured meal preparation but also witness the potential for variety within the AFBI framework. By dividing the plan into two batches, the cookbook recognizes the importance of preventing monotony while maintaining a balanced and energizing routine.

In essence, the AFBI Diet Cookbook for Beginners is a guide to fostering a mindful, anti-inflammatory, and balanced relationship with food. It's an invitation to explore new flavors, embrace nutritional diversity, and embark on a journey towards sustained well-being. As individuals savor the delectable recipes within these pages, they are not just nourishing their bodies; they are embracing a lifestyle that promotes balance, energy, and overall vitality. May this cookbook be a source of inspiration, guiding you on a path to a healthier and more fulfilling life. Cheers to your wellness journey with the AFBI Diet!

My Valued Reader,

I trust this culinary journey has not only ignited your passion for wholesome eating but has also become a haven of inspiration, solace, and invaluable insights. Each carefully curated recipe within this the complete AFBI Diet Cookbook for Beginners reflects a dedication to excellence, with a profound understanding of the comprehensive guide to the glycemic index diet.

Crafted with meticulous attention to detail, these recipes go beyond the realm of mere sustenance; they are a testament to the art of nourishing the body and soul. Your reviews, experiences, and insights are treasures that guide me on this culinary odyssey.

Every evaluation is a stepping stone for refinement, as I aspire to tailor this cookbook to surpass your expectations. Let's engage in a dialogue that transcends the pages, creating a connection that resonates with your culinary preferences and well-being goals.

Warm Culinary Regards,

# Tina Feldman